10

SECONDS

THAT

CHANGED

MY

LIFE

IAIN M. MACLEOD

Paperback ISBN: 9781946824394
Hardback ISBN: 9781946824400
Ebook ISBN: 9781946824417
Audio CD ISBN: 9781946824424
Audio mp3 ISBN: 9781946824431
LCCN: 2019932468

Audiobook Production: ProAudioVoices | www.proaudiovoices.com
Audiobook Narration: Toni Frutin | www.tonifrutin.com
Editing, Design: Janet Angelo | www.designindiego.com

Names: MacLeod, Iain M., 1963-, author.
Title: 10 seconds that changed my life / Iain M. MacLeod.
Description: [Florida] : IndieGo Publishing, 2019. | Summary: This first-person account interspersed with original poetry charts the various stages of the author's hospital experience and personal journey through joy and sorrow, frustration and elation, and the reality of coming home to a new normal.
Identifiers: LCCN 2019932468 | ISBN 9781946824400 (hardcover) | ISBN 9781946824394 (pbk.) | ISBN 9781946824417 (ebook) | ISBN 9781946824424 (Audio CD) | ISBN 9781946824431 (mp3)
Subjects: LCSH: MacLeod, Iain M. – 1963 -. | People with disabilities -- Great Britain -- Biography. | People with disabilities – Scotland – Personal narratives. | Scotland -- Poetry. | BISAC: BIOGRAPHY & AUTOBIOGRAPHY / Medical. | POETRY / General. | SOCIAL SCIENCE / People   with Disabilities.
Classification: LCC PR6113.A254 T46 2019 (print) | LCC PR6113.A254 (ebook) | DDC 920.M33--dc23
LC record available at https://lccn.loc.gov/2019932468

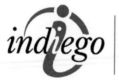

PUBLISHING
Our Brilliance . Your Success
WWW.INDIEGOPUBLISHING.COM
WWW.INDIEGOPUBLISHING.CO.UK
WWW.GETINDIEGO.COM

DEDICATION

I dedicate this book to my parents, whose love and support have seen me through this ordeal.

ACKNOWLEDGMENTS

I would like to sincerely thank everyone who helped me during my illness and recovery: Mr. and Mrs. Paterson, Mr. and Mrs. McPherson, Fochabers Medical Practice, The Moray Council (Social Services), NHS Grampian Hospitals; Dr. Greys, Elgin; Aberdeen Royal Infirmary (ARI); Woodend Hospital (NRU), Aberdeen and Turner Memorial, Keith; Wheelchair Service (MARS), Aberdeen; my Mum and Dad for their love and support over the months; my sisters Anne and Eileen for their support, and especially Anne and her husband Steven. Special thanks to Janet Angelo for her thoughtful editing of this book and for her friendship, and to Toni Frutin for her lovely narration of the audiobook.

CHAPTERS

———————

10

SECONDS

THAT

CHANGED

MY

LIFE

CHAPTER 1

Not an Ordinary Day

Thursday, 15th June, 2017, will be forever embedded in my brain as the day my life changed. I never could have imagined to what extent. The day started as every other day, but it would prove to be anything but an ordinary day. I would end the day lying in Intensive Care in an Aberdeen hospital with a ventilating tube down my throat.

I awoke at home that morning about the usual time, 6:00 a.m. The dawn chorus was singing merrily. I groped under the pillow to locate the controller that opens the door and blinds, turns on the lights, and switches on the TV and radio. Measuring about ten by five by three centimeters, I hung it around my neck with a black bootlace, turned down the duvet, and moved to get out of bed. Usually, I put on Radio Scotland each morning to find out the latest news, but for some strange reason, on that particular morning, I did not switch on the radio. Probably thought I would switch it on while sitting at the table having my first coffee of the day in about ten minutes.

A few months earlier, I had bought a memory foam mattress because the old mattress was sagging in the middle. On hindsight, it would prove to be the worst thing I ever bought.

Rolling out of bed onto my knees that morning, which I did because the mattress was low to the floor, my left elbow slipped on the memory foam protector and wedged between the bed and the bedside cabinet. The morning before, my left hand slid off the mattress, and I had the passing thought, *I must remember to move that cabinet today.* I wish I had remembered!

With my elbow wedged, I tried to heave my torso off the bed and onto the floor, but I did not have the strength. I lay strewn across the bed, right arm lying on the mattress at about one o'clock and the left wedged, palm against the cabinet and elbow against the side of the bed, my legs splayed open like pincers on the floor.

I was well and truly trapped.

I remember thinking, *How am I going to get out of this mess?* The pain in my left arm was extremely severe, like no pain I had experienced before. I wriggled to free my arm, but it was jammed tight. Then, I had the bright idea of lowering my wedged elbow down to the floor through the space between the cabinet and bed because that would allow me to get onto my knees and hoist myself to a standing position using my elbow crutches.

Centimeter by centimeter, my elbow slid down. At this point, I actually thought my idea would work, but my elbow came to a sudden stop halfway down where the mattress meets the base of the bed and there were a few millimeters cap. My bright idea did not work. In fact, it was going to prove an extremely bad idea. Instead of working its way loose, my elbow became more deeply lodged between the bed and the bedside cabinet.

Now I was well and truly trapped. Lying half sprawled across the mattress, half on the floor, I felt the fight for life slowly ebbing with every wriggle. The controller hung around my neck, but I could not reach it. I could not free myself.

Minutes turned into hours. As the hours passed, I felt myself falling into a sleep-haze, though I never lost consciousness. Unfortunately, I vividly remember everything through that infernally long time. This was going to be a long wait for help, if it ever arrived. The pain in my left shoulder was excruciating.

I resigned myself to the fact that I was going to die in that room, and felt strangely peaceful. Dying in my house in my beloved Fochabers was a comforting thought. I have done many things in life, but never thought the end would come with a simple thing such as getting out of bed. My mind turned to my mother. She would be totally devastated and would never get over it. I imagined the police telling my parents and their reaction. How utterly, inconsolably distraught she would be. I would have done anything rather than put my mother through that pain.

I lay trapped for eight hours. My body was starting to shut down. The pain in my left arm began to ease, and my breathing slowed.

Mum and Dad were on holiday in the campervan. Mum always phones every morning to find out how I am each day. The phone rang three times, but it was under the pillow, out of reach. Each time Dad left a message. When I didn't answer, he phoned my neighbours, Charlie and Minnie Paterson, who had a key, to ask if they could check to see if everything was okay. They told me later they had noticed that my blinds, which were normally open by mid-morning, were still closed. Suddenly, I heard a key in the lock, and the door opened, and Charlie and Minnie appeared in the bedroom doorway and said they would phone an ambulance. Five minutes passed, though it might have been longer, and my GP Dr. Critchley appeared by my side.

"Hello, Iain," she said in a soothing, comforting voice. She examined me. I was told later that I had only fifteen minutes to live if I had not been found. A short time later, two paramedics appeared at the bedroom door. They extracted me and took an ECG trace of my heart. I was put into a chair and wheeled down the ramp to the waiting ambulance. Being wheeled out of the house, passing through the short hallway with its framed photograph of Stornoway Harbour (marking the maiden voyage of the new ferry, *Isle of Lewis*), down the ramp and past my silver car, my pride and joy, little did I know that I probably would never drive again.

In the ambulance, I was transferred to a stretcher and strapped in like an Egyptian mummy. On the journey to Dr. Gray's hospital in Elgin, about ten miles away, I remember thinking, as I passed the landmarks of my beloved Fochabers, *See you again soon!*

At the hospital, in Accident and Emergency, the doctors and nurses fussed over me like worker ants going about their daily routines. They examined me and took my vital signs. I remember speaking to them as I lay on the examining bed – not about the state of the world, though it had a lot to be desired, nor philosophical conversation, but answering their numerous questions. That would be the last time that I would ever speak in my voice again. Something that I had taken for granted for fifty years was gone now, never to return.

CHAPTER 2

Rude Awakening

"Hello, Iain. You've been asleep for fourteen hours." The nurse spoke in a soothing voice. I gradually woke from my slumber. As I did so, I became aware of a tube down my throat and a machine in front of me flashing multi-coloured lights. Where was I? What had happened? My eyes darted about the room taking in my surroundings. I felt confused and frightened, alone and scared. I wanted my mum to hold my hand, wipe my brow and say everything was okay.

Instead, I was alone and scared. When my brain adjusted to the surroundings, I began to piece together the events of that day, and slowly realised what had happened. I would have liked having a nurse or doctor sit by my bedside to explain what had happened and where I was. When I was lucid, the nurse told me I was in Intensive Care at the Aberdeen Royal Infirmary (ARI). She said that I was rushed from Elgin to

Aberdeen, a trip of sixty miles, in a 'blue lighter' ambulance with a doctor onboard. The consultant told my parents that they thought I wouldn't survive, the second time that I was near death's door within twenty-four hours.

As I lay on my right-hand side, my eyes scanned the room. I could see eight to ten beds in the ward. A nurses' station stood about three meters directly in front of my room. A wall of glass bathed the ward with natural light. Sliding doors opened when a ferry-type boat, which the ward rested upon, reached the concrete ramp.

Why the ward lay on a boat, I could never figure out.

I was not allowed to drink, as I was 'nil by mouth.' I was allowed 'lollipops,' not the sweet treats I imagined when I first heard them described as such. They were sponges on sticks dipped in water, and only meant to moisten your mouth, but I was always getting a row for squeezing the sponge in my mouth to taste the water and suck the sponge dry. I was not allowed to swallow as I had a bad swallow, whatever that meant.

One hot day, when I was lying on my back, I spied a glass of water from the corner of my eye and started fantasizing how good it would be to drink. How beautiful the cold water would feel in my mouth, the soothing chill of liquid going down my throat into my stomach.

Hours later I would be off on the next adventure in this surreal world that had become my life.

The florescent lights in the bright corridor flashed by as I was whisked along on the trolley.

Within twenty-four hours of being admitted to Intensive Care, I was on the way to the surgical theatre with a blood clot in my leg. I recall speaking to the theatre nurses and being transferred onto the bed from the trolley. I mumbled something to the surgeon before she injected a pre-anesthetic in my wrist, which heralded a mask being placed over my nose and mouth. Counting back from ten, I reached six, and the next thing I remember, I was waking up in Intensive Care. My upper leg was bandaged, and a drain ran into a plastic bag that rested on the floor next to my bed. I experienced morphine dreams like I had never dreamt before, surreal dreams that were so vivid they seemed real. In one dream, I was sitting on the ceiling of a lift looking down on all the people in it. The second dream involved metal storage units. I was walking between the containers and saw friends along the sidelines.

Lying in the bed one day was very much the same as the next. I soon got used to the ward's routine and recognised the various nurses who looked after me. Intensive Care is one nurse to one patient. My view was slightly restricted because I had a tube down my throat that attached to a machine next to my bed. As long as I had that ventilating tube down my throat, I did not let my mum come to visit, as I didn't want her to see me like that. Dad always asked if I wanted to see Mum, but I shook my head furiously.

The doctors did their ward rounds three times a day. After introducing themselves, they had a group meeting at the end of my bed. I have taken some courses in human physiology, so I listened to their whispered conversations with interest. Often, I did not agree with them, and shook my head in silent protest. Slowly their whispers became positive. They were all nice, but one young doctor, very kind and pleasant, knelt by my bedside after a group meeting and said that I was getting a couple of tubes out. I nodded in delight, and wanted to shout "Thank goodness!" The next day two tubes came out, but another went in. This time a thinner yellow tube was inserted up my nose and down into my stomach. The doctor tried inserting up the right nostril without any luck, so up the left nostril it went.

An X-ray was taken to find out if the tube had reached its target. It had not! The doctor tried again up the left nostril and another X-ray was taken. Success!

The vocal cords lie on the left of the nasal passage, and by inserting the tube up the left nostril, this can damage the right cord. My voice was not great before I went into hospital, but having the tube inserted up my left nostril and kept in for seven weeks could possibly damage the right cord. My voice would be damaged for life, so the tubes must stay in only for the short term, a week or ten days, before being removed and a PEG inserted into the stomach. I got my PEG seven weeks later.

By the end of the process, it felt like I'd had enough food down my tube to last a year, but it was probably only enough for a month or so. It was a shock to my mum seeing her son lying listless on the trolley. I did not really understand what was happening. At the end of the food manufacturing time, I was transferred to another trolley and wheeled back to the ward where I was transferred to my bed, and a drip was set up by the bedside to give me my first meal since being admitted into Intensive Care. The nurse let me smell the delicious meal, and I was very glad I was 'nil by mouth!' It was a pale-yellow liquid in a bag, about 250 ml. I was told that it contained all the nutrients and fibre that my body needed. A clear tube ran from the hanging bag to a tube in my nose. The liquid dripped into a small plastic holding container before making its way down the tube and into my stomach.

Being fed twice a day, morning and evening, I soon got used to the times the bags were put up. In a strange way, I looked forward to this daily ritual. Life followed its usual uneventful routines; one day was pretty much the same as the next. I stayed in Intensive Care for two weeks before moving to my next ward.

CHAPTER 3

Don't Diss Me, I'm Able

I have been disabled, a life member of the club, since the age of three following a flu epidemic in 1966 while my family lived in Stornoway, an island off the West Coast of Scotland. I suffer from Cerebral Palsy. The medical profession love to put everyone into a box and give them a label to hang around their neck. I came under the umbrella of Cerebral Palsy, and I basked under that umbrella for fifty-plus years without any major crisis except for a few scares, until now when my world had been turned upside down and might never be the same again, all because of a slippery mattress cover.

I grew up in Moray, where my dad got a job with the North-East Water Board, as it was called then. My childhood was good and full of memories. One over-riding memory is the fun I had on my tricycle. It was good exercise to keep my legs supple. Mum would strap my feet into the pedals, and away I would go for about an hour or so, cycling around Lhanbryde.

I went to a special school, as they were called then. There were varied educational abilities, but the teachers all did their best. If I were a child today, I would go to a mainstreamed school, but the world was a different place then. Procrastinating pseudo-professionals ruled the day with their Freudian, idealised utter nonsense.

—◦◦◦—

Old School Yard

Boarded up the stone building weathers
Not revealing past years of educational achievements
People who stop unaware of childhood dreams
Abandoned and vacant and neglected
Unknowing testament of a forgotten past

Children played and laughed together and loved
Not caring of the world and its introspective harshness
Unaware of life's multiplicity of layered carpeting
Labelled chained boxes of physical imperfections
Lifelong barriers to overcome of unfilled aspirations
Those were the days of untarnished minds
Unconcerned and carefree childhoods
Unknowing of the world that lay beyond
Unconscious of what the future may hold
How the labelled boxes would shape and determine.

Days of uncluttered purity and innocent childhood
Distant remembrances in a sterile environment
Decades pass, memories become transient
Old adages of imbecilic slowly diminishing
Memories fade as downward slope looms
Old school yard gradually fades in the mists of time

~w~

PMR

Princess Margaret Rose Hospital, restorer of life
Princess Margaret Rose, daughter of King George IV
Southside of Edinburgh
The seriously ill child lay helpless and dying

Asian flu assigning the child to the lifelong club
Succumbing to societal vagaries and patronisation
Life's badge for being different in a perfect world
Slowly and painfully, he recovered
Endured operation after operation
Body crafted and molded to semi-perfection
Mr. Fulford rebuilt and crafted and restored
Surgical skills artistry shaped the sculpture

Life's path divided and the one less travelled trundled
Swaying from side to side, the turns undulated
A world of stereotype nothing objects
Educated to below par was the 'normal' expectation
Overcoming hurdles proved to be a lifetime occupation

Perceived normality was never an option
In a world of perfection and flawless purities
The downward spiral question's the point of life

—ᴧᴧ—

Stornoway Gael

Madainn mhath and Feasgar math
Gaelic phrases of my youth
In a land of ancient tradition and cleared people
Sheep over people

I lie in the sofa bed, in a Laxdale living room, watching
the magenta skyline
Watching, through the four paneled windows, the
sodium silhouette of Stornoway
Land of my nostalgic reminiscences and pride
Berthed Cullivan ready to return to Ullapool
Right lies Stornoway Castle standing guard over the
island

Laxdale, a few miles north of Stornoway
Up the cluthan and to the right
Tar roofed white cottage with lovingly crafted peat
stack
Long days cutting peats at Loch Crinabhat
Eaten alive by midges
Tea made from ice-cold well water, best ever
Crackan biscuits, hard insides and brown outer

Superbly delicious with butter and jam
An anticipated treat

Recollections of a bygone age
Brown corrugated cowshed at the bottom of the croft
Once a sanctuary of bovine activity
Now a refuse for feral kittens

Walking down the starran for adventures
Green wire-messed gate; end of a stony dirt track
Protection from the outside world

Running down the croft
Before becoming a member of the lifelong club
Asian flu robbing a boy of his childhood and adulthood

Instead succumbing to societal vagaries
Relatives reminding of this loss
"I remember when...!" only served to frustrate
Early years of forgotten blankness

Now, on the downward spiral, a time to reflect
Long summers of distant memories
Rose tinted views of idealism and utopian perfection
Though it might not have been
The desire to go back to Stornoway does not appeal
Reminiscences are historical recollections of the past
Always will be proud of being a Gael and of my
heritage

Callanish Stones

A land shrouded in mystical and ancient past
People worshipped celestial gods
Offerings of appeasement ritually offered
To improve body or receive spiritual forgiveness

Callias respectful of their ancient inhabitants
Stone circle in praise of astronomical wonderment
The village courteously gracious of centuries past
Their achievements and pious reverence worshipped

Stones of past civilisation erected in homage
Their mystical significance remains lost in time
Ancestral ancestors impregnate my DNA
My time capsule to the past lies biologically hidden
The lineage will end with me

After leaving school, I went to Beaumont College in Lancaster for a couple of years. There, I learned how to look after myself doing daily tasks such as cooking and washing. Upon coming back home, I realised I needed to pass my driving test so I could achieve my ambitions, so I set about this challenge with determination. After passing my driving test, I started the process of re-educating myself by attending Adult Basic Education classes, going to the local college and being a mature student. In the early nineties, I joined The Open University and remain a committed OU student. I eventually attained a postgraduate standard of education. When I lived on my own in my beloved Fochabers, I used elbow crutches and a wheelchair for mobility and was furiously independent. I had only one carer, who came in ninety minutes a week to do housework. That all changed following my accident. One of the things I had quickly to get used to was being hoisted in a sling before I could do anything, hoisted into my wheelchair, and rolled left and right so the nurses could get the sling underneath my body.

To say I was comfortable with this would be lying, and I never will be. By far the biggest thing I had to accept and be relaxed with was personal care. This can be very awkward. Having someone help you with the most basic of bodily functions is so embarrassing. To make it worse, if that person is thirty-plus years your junior and the opposite sex, it can feel so undignified, though the nurses were all very professional and never thought anything about it.

No matter how often someone helps me with personal care, I always feel so uncomfortable, probably because I am so independent, and never needed personal care before the Wedged Elbow Incident, a day that will go down in infamy. This is why I am finding it difficult to fully come to terms with someone else looking after me.

I have been patronised all my life, and it has never bothered me; it is part and parcel of being different in a gloss-covered perfect world. The fact I was in a wheelchair and spoke more slowly than most people meant I was fair game to be spoken to very precisely, as if I couldn't comprehend, though I could, or shouted at, as if I couldn't hear, though my hearing was perfectly normal. After all, I was physically disabled; surely, I had trouble understanding, right? Not right!

Now, since the Elbow Incident, my breathing and speech are more laboured, which means the patronising has gotten worse.

-√w√-

Patronising Perceptions

The figure sits in his own small world
Bereft of sense and rationality and neuronal connections
How graciously society bestows accolades

Readily the crown of physical imperfections honoured
Broca's damage just adds to the imbecilic patronising
Retardation and disability is causally linked insinuated

Educated to just write their names
"After all, that's all they will need," the 'professionals'
procrastinate
Preaching Freudian misguided nonsense
In a world of psychological bombastic bureaucrats

The old school mentality continues in ridiculousness
The figure sits thinking of his thesis and possibilities
Lost in his own world of higher educational attainment
Higher than the procrastinating professionals
Who want to take the praise and credit
Personal endeavour and fulfilment the only driving
force

～w～

Sanctimonious Hypocrisy

Geocentrically orbiting the Earth rotationally
Milky Way of infinite empty space
Revolving ball of humanity and caring sanctuary

A World of self-righteous duplicity and perfection
Hypocritical flawless impurities and puritanism
The latest teabag or the unseasonality of the weather
Designed to show the simplicity of character

Subliminal Darwinism is purposely disguised
Survival of the fittest ensures differentiation continues
Denial rigorously refuted with epitaph proportionality

The world continues to spin on its axis
Caring do-gooders continue to speak new teabags
Simplistic patronisation judged on Brocial appearance
Spontaneity will never be without character familiarity
Species propagation potentially and superiority

CHAPTER 4

The Grand Hospital Tour

The paintings flashed past like scenes from a train window. I was in another zone. The next ward was something similar to Intensive Care, but instead of one nurse looking after me, I now had two. It was a big ward split in two by a white wooden partition. My bed was in a corner with a locker to the right of it. Behind the bed was a window that looked over Aberdeen Harbour. It was early July, and the days were mostly fine, so the window was open most days. The window was higher than the bed, so I could not see out or even adjust myself to see out. I could not move let alone get out of bed even if I wanted to, but I enjoyed smelling the sea air and hearing the sounds of the harbour. The ward was hot, so any fresh air was most welcome.

Visits from my parents and sister were important at this time, as I was still trying to come to terms with the enormity of my situation. To see familiar faces was such a morale booster that it instantly improved my spirits. One thing I do remember of those days was the evening my feeding tube came out of my nose. The young doctor tried to re-insert it again up my left nostril. I distinctly remember him saying, as he was poised to ram the tube up my hooter, "This might be a bit uncomfortable." A bit! He failed! Handing the tube to a colleague, he mumbled something about letting him have a go. That young doctor also failed. At this stage my nose felt like a wide tunnel, and I half expected them to run down Union Street inviting the public to have a go at shoving the feeding tube up my nose! Seriously, I think all medical students should experience a feeding tube being inserted up their nose. This would let them have an insight into how a patient might feel when the procedure is done incorrectly.

I then spent a few days in the renal ward, as my kidneys were not functioning properly either, before going on my travels again. I got a single room that looked onto different corridors that went to various parts of the hospital. The room was about three meters long by two meters wide. On the ceiling was a track hoist with a double hoisting mechanism. Directly in front of me was an en suite bathroom with a sliding door.

A small groove in the door's track meant a patient could be hoisted from their bed through to the shower in the bathroom. I was too sore to have a shower and had bed-baths instead.

My days were mostly filled with watching people hurry back and forth. The nurses came in at different times of the day to see me and perform some task or medical procedure, or to take my vital signs.

My arms were very sore and rested on pillows. As my voice was weak and my arms were useless appendages attached to my shoulders, I could not call for the nurses. A system was devised whereby I attracted their attention by shaking my head when they passed the open door. This worked to a certain extent, but not if they didn't bother looking at me as they hurried by. Still, it was better than nothing.

⌁⌁⌁

Vistas pasted like scenes from a speeding train through the countryside. My next port of call was neurology. 'Welcome to Neuroscience,' the sign said, as I emerged from the lift, There lay the cruel irony, as before I ended up in hospital, I was going to study for my PhD in neuroscience. I stayed in neurology for the rest of my time in the ARI other than ten days in the High Dependency Unit (HDU).

The ward was a temporary accommodation until their actual abode was modernised. It was a busy ward. At first, I was put into a room with four beds. At least the windows opened, but the ward was stifling during the day with the afternoon sun streaming in. These sauna-like conditions persisted throughout the evenings as well. My health had not improved greatly by this stage either; my left arm was very sore, and the right, although not as sore, was painful. They both rested on pillows. I could not speak too well because of the feeding tube coming out of my nose like a swinging elephant's trunk. When I needed a nurse, my roommates called for one, which was good of them. The window was too high to see out of from the bed, but when I was raised so the nurses could perform some task or other, I saw that the ward looked out onto a car park.

Meal times were problematic because I was still 'nil by mouth,' and watching my fellow patients tuck into whatever they ordered made my food cravings even worse. Watching them drink cups of coffee was sheer torture. It was seven long weeks before I was allowed coffee. When that glorious day came, a lovely young Irish lady from the Speech and Language department gave me the warm, aromatic nectar. Getting my first coffee in weeks was such a great feeling that it must rank high in life's achievements. A week later, my health took a turn for the worse, and I was moved to the observations ('obs') department of the neurology ward.

There were about five or so beds in 'obs.' My bed was moved directly in front of the nurses' station so they could watch me. I got to know the nurses and when they would be on duty. During this time, the ward physiotherapists hoisted me into a high-backed wheelchair to allow me to sit for a brief period each day.

During these times, I often reminisced about my happy life in Fochabers.

CHAPTER 5

Ode to Fochabers

I lived happily in Fochabers, a delightful town in the North-East of Scotland, for seventeen years until June 2017 when my whole life fell apart. I had hoped and believed I would be there until the end of my days. I was well known in the community, and participated in village life. The prospect of leaving Fochabers, possibly never living there again, made me so very sad, especially because of a ten-second silly accident. I loved my house, and the adaptations made it suitable and special.

~w~

Fochabers

Driving away that Friday night heralded a new chapter
Late September weather transition merged
Friday night Fochabers, Saturday Inverness

Not realising the empathetic pull of the village
Bonds deepen over the rolling years

House crafted and tailored to suit
Doors marked are characteristics of hidden happiness
Satisfaction of ecstasy a gauge of blissful contentment
Contented dwelling is testament of pride and fulfilment
Unconscious realisation of singleton reality

Wheeled freedom represents solitude tranquility
Aimlessly chaired wandering naturally rejuvenates
Physical barriers of normal chains are briefly broken

The northeast village unaware of personal happiness
Spinning striped recognition being inner contentment
In a world of uncertainty and insecurity
Fochabers restores clarity and peaceful satisfaction

The Spey a source of great joyous pleasure
Looking down the undulating waters of restoration
Calming qualities of tranquility soothingly washes
In an act of contemplative meditation
A neural confusion to placid peacefulness

~\/\~

I used to love wandering around the village exploring
scenic walks. My favourite spot was looking down The
Spey, a source of great solace, peace and tranquility. I

used to spend a lot of time at the Memorial Gardens gazing at The Spey flowing past. There is a bench on the grassy bank to invite people to sit and gaze at the river. I loved sitting next to it in my electric wheelchair. (A log that had separated the grass from the path was taken away so that I had a better view of the river.) That bench inspired me to write the poem "The Seat" in this book, as I wondered one day how many people sat on that bench looking at the same view that I loved. On nice summer days, I enjoyed watching kayaks and canoes meandering down the river.

While nomadically zooming about the village, I was thinking of assignments and how to phrase essays or theses. When I was studying for my MSc (all those stress-free hours!), my itinerant lifestyle helped concentrate my mind. Talking to people made the world a nicer place and washed the cares of the day away. I miss having conversations with people in the village and visiting my usual places. Happiness is often the simple things in life, which cannot be replaced with coldness and sensibility, rationality and wrongly perceived ideas of society's 'we know what's best for you' attitude uttered by those who should know better but often don't.

Now, as I am embarking on my PhD, I will not have my beloved Fochabers to restore my calm tranquility and The Spey for academic inspiration. Whilst it is true that you can't eat scenery, as I have heard said, there's more to life than rational puritanism. Looking at calming scenery is good for a person's physical and psychological well-being.

-ᴟᴝᴟ-

Autumn Colours

Crimson reds and oranges and rustic browns and
lemony yellow interspersed in a lime canopy
A wall of multi-coloured leaves
A waterfall of hued descending leaves

Multi-coloured branches
Guardians of remembrance stones of loved ones
departed
Overlooking the Spey
Reassurance of the flowing waters
White horses cascading to form swirls

Water glints in autumn sun
Falling from the sky like leaves falling from trees
Blanketed soil in readiness for next spring's birth

-ᴟᴝᴟ-

I loved Fochabers with all my heart like I have never
loved any place before. I participated in village activities
and spent money locally. I talked with everyone I met,
and I could never nip to the shop without chatting with
people along the way. I would do my shopping, go back
home, and be back ten minutes later because I had

forgotten something, usually milk, and the assistants would say with big smiles as I entered the shop, "What have you forgotten this time?"

-∿-

Belly Clock

Standing guard with reassuring presence since 1798
On the hour every hour the time booms out
Reverberating near and far
Performing a valuable information service

Steadfastly booming out its hourly prompt
Reminder of an appointment or catching a bus
Timekeeping for activities of daily importance
Or just a gentle reminder of the hours passing

The clock is a focal feature of daily life
Witness to triumph and sadness
A bystander to days of wedding celebrations
Sad departing souls of the great and good
Every facet of village life throughout the years

-∿-

Fountain Focality

Commemorating water to Fochabers in 1798
The fountain is a prominent feature

Focal point for all to see and admire
Obvious treasure for locals and tourists alike
Sitting transfixed in wonderment
Whiling the time away in mesmerising tranquility
A landmark and point of reference for placement

A conspicuous symbiotic marriage with the clock
Standing guard over the village in an angel-like way
Cascading water symbolises cleansing from high
Architectural details of past craftsmanship is a legacy
Five cherubs make sure all is well as guardian angels

Commemoration has become guardianship,
For all to see and admire adoringly in forbearance,
Lasting inheritance of remembrance from the past.

∿

The Seat

Picture framed between trees
Overlooking the Spey as it flows past
Rod fishing for salmon forms the migratory dance
Canoes weaving their way eastward

The seat is witness to all habitation of the Spey
Exposed to all the elements from baking heat to snow
Patiently waiting for its next passing viewer to sit

Generations finding solitude and comfort

Retired GPs to Londoners seeking Scottish romance
All searching for inner peace
All lost in contemplative pondering
Admiring the picturesque scenes

Mind drifting and reflecting
Troubles being washed and purified
Amidst the uninterrupted continuous water
Reflecting on life's strangeness and tragic woes
Finding calm and peace and inner tranquility

Glassic-Gibbon wrote, "The land endures…"
And the seat endures
Restoring rationality and peacefulness
Unknowingly the river surges past on its journey
Unaware of its rejuvenating harmonious serenity

~w~

Even though traveling in my mind was a pleasant distraction as I whiled away the hours, I was beginning to find my hospital stay very boring, as one day was the same as the next. I longed for some mental stimulus and wanted a game of chess. Julia and Megan, ward physiotherapists, took on the case and acquired a travelling chess set and numbered it for me, as I was having trouble speaking. In the end, I found it easier to nod at the piece I wanted moved. Eventually an opponent was found and a time was arranged. I won in four moves.

CHAPTER 6

Back "Home" in Neurology

As the days became weeks, my health fluctuated from feeling better to getting worse. This meant I was moved back and forth from 'obs' to a single room. One of the times I was in a single room, I was coughing badly and was diagnosed as suffering from a hospital acquired infection. A thin white plastic tube was inserted up the right nostril and down my throat to clear phlegm, which was gathering there because I was finding it difficult to cough up. I was moved to the High Dependency Unit (HDU) and put on a course of antibiotics to treat the infection.

The first thing they did was to insert needles in my neck and wrist, quite painless – aye, right! – attached to tube lines that monitored my heart rate. At night, a fan was trained on my upper body to decrease my high temperature.

While in HDU, I got rid of that awful feeding tube from my nose, and a PEG was inserted directly into my stomach. I was not completely clear of the chest infection, and while the PEG was inserted, I coughed, spluttered and writhed through the entire ordeal. The procedure involved inserting a laparoscopic camera down my throat (that was painful), and making an incision on the upper skin to locate precisely where the PEG would be inserted, after which a clear tube was pushed into the stomach, a valve put over the end, and a linking tube from where the feeding tube was attached.

The whole procedure took about twenty minutes, and I returned to 'obs' in neurology where I had left five days previously.

I was getting on well with PEG. At least I had got rid of that horrible tube hanging down from my nose, but seven days later, at 11:00 p.m., I started coughing up blood. It was as if someone was saying, "You haven't suffered enough. Here, try this for size!" Clare, the nurse, was amazing in her calm handling of the situation as my vital signs fell. My sister, who was on holiday in the caravan, was phoned at about 1:00 a.m. in case I might die this time. I was taken to theatre at about 1:10 a.m.

"See you in a few days," a nurse said to me as I left the ward.

I remember speaking to the surgeon about drinking coffee; as a bet, he had given up for week or a month (I can't remember which), and he won.

The mask went over my nose, and counting backwards from ten, I got to six.

Next thing I remember, I was waking up in HDU. I was almost clear of the chest infection, but would go into fits of coughing occasionally, so the nurse offered to insert a thinner tube up my hooter and down my throat to suction out the phlegm. I declined the offer, as I did not want another tube up my nose.

I stayed in HDU for two days and one night before being moved back to the neurology ward. I did not sleep well that night, as I was not allowed my sleeping tablet. They discovered I had a bacterium in my urine that was antibiotic resistant – just to add to everything else I had! This meant I had to be isolated from the other patients, so for the remaining time I spent in neurology, I was in single rooms except when I spent time in 'obs.'

I got quite bored on my own with only the radio for company. All the rooms were roughly the same. They had windows on the back wall that looked onto a car park. Toilets just inside the door as you walked into the room. Wardrobe and sink on the far wall.

When I was in the larger ward with several beds, my fellow patients called for assistance if I needed a nurse, but in a single room, I was on my own. My arms were still very sore, the left sorer than the right, and rested on pillows. As a result, I did not have the strength to push the buzzer to call for a nurse.

The ward occupational therapist saw this as a big problem and went off to find an alarm I could use. She came back one day with a large red circular object.

Measuring about seven centimeters across, it was certainly noticeable! It was an extra sensitive nurse call alarm. Positioned under my right thumb, I had just enough strength to push the red button. I was forever accidently pushing the button whenever I moved in bed, and the nurses would come running. The red buzzer was associated with me to such an extent that when I came back to neurology from HDU, a search began to locate it and get the red button back to me from the room I had left two days before. Even the doctors wondered where it was and helped in the search.

It was mid-July, so it was sunny most days and the windows were open, but it was Aberdeen, so the rain was never far away. Some days the mornings were beautiful sunshine, and I would foolishly think it was going to be a nice day, but by afternoon there were hailstorms.

Sometimes I asked the nurses to raise the bed so I could look out the window to ease the boredom. Looking at the passing cars, I wondered if the people in them were visitors coming to see relatives or friends at the hospital, or hospital workers.

The hospital had a Patients' Garden where I loved going when someone pushed me. It was a serene place with flowerbeds and aromatic shrubs. In the middle of the garden was a shelter from the elements, if required. It was a new garden and not yet officially opened.

The whole place was well thought out: wide walkways, seats at just the right height, and an automatic door to make entrance and exit easier for wheelchair users.

I loved going there to forget my situation for a while. It meant I could get out of the ward for an hour or two, but far more importantly, I could get fresh air into my lungs. If the ward physiotherapists had time in the afternoons, they took me to the garden; otherwise, it was Mum and Dad.

I always enjoyed my time in the garden.

-ᴡᴡ-

Buzzing Bonanza

The bee methodically circles, buzzing from plant to plant
A ritualistic dance passed down the generations
Orbiting the flowers with precision probing
Gathering the sweet nectar for storage

Focused on the task it was born
Single-minded unwavering
Concentrating on its mission
Obtaining nutritious nectar for the next generation

Next generation methodically circles
The genetic cycle of probing passes to the next

-ᴡᴡ-

The garden was on the roof of one of the buildings, and I enjoyed watching through the safety glass wall the arriving and departing ambulances from Accident and Emergency. A couple meters inside the hospital from the garden was a quiet room that I loved for its serenity. It was a beautiful space with stained glass windows and comfortable seating, a lovely place to be alone and recharge one's batteries.

It was a sunny day when I celebrated my fifty-fourth birthday. First time I celebrated a birthday in hospital. The ward was so kind giving me a card and a cake, but since I was nil by mouth, I could not eat a piece of the cake, though Mum and Dad enjoyed it.

During my stay in neurology, I used an alphabet board to communicate, as my voice was not strong enough by this stage. The alphabet board was often a source of amusement because of misspellings and unintended meanings because I was unable to write in the proper context.

While speaking to one of the auxiliaries, I happened to mention that I enjoyed listening to heavy metal music. Upon hearing this, Liam recorded, in his own time and on his iPod Nano, heavy metal for me to listen to while he was on duty, and left me contentedly head-banging to Iron Maiden.

Lying in the bed on a humid July night, one song in particular stuck in my mind: "Empire of the Clouds." That song will always be special to me, and will evoke happy memories of my time in neurology. I will never forget Liam's exceptional kindness.

Months later, when Liam and his girlfriend came to visit me in Keith, he told me an amusing story. When he put the earphones in my ears for the first time, I was head banging to Iron Maiden so hard that the bed was shaking. A nurse asked Liam if I was feeling okay because she thought I was having a seizure!

~vw~

The machine made a terrible noise as I underwent a serious of tests to determine what exactly was wrong. So much blood was taken that I thought there would not be enough left for me! Nothing out of the ordinary was seen in the red fluid. Then came the washing machines. Magnetic resonance imaging (MRI) and computer tomography (CT) were taken. A CT scan was done when the doctors suspected I had a chest infection. An MRI revealed nothing significant. A lumbar puncture was taken. That was a pleasant experience – not! The procedure involves a needle being inserted into the fourth/fifth vertebrae in the spine and a few drops of cerebrospinal fluid (CSF) taken. This was done twice as the first time did not work. It revealed nothing out of the ordinary. The last test was examining the muscles in my arms to find out if they were functioning properly. A needle electrode was prodded up and down my left arm and readings taken. My right arm was tested for comparison. This showed quite a lot of peripheral muscle damage in my left arm compared to my right. The doctor said my arms should heal in time. I was glad to hear this good news and could see light at the end of the tunnel. Things looked a bit more promising than at the start of the testing process.

In late August, Penny and her colleagues of the Speech and Language Team allowed me to drink my first coffee in eight weeks! The warm aromatic liquid had never tasted so good as it did that day. It was great to finally be able to eat, but I do not mean solid food; that would be weeks away. No, my food was yoghurt, yoghurt and more yoghurt, three times a day, morning, noon and night. I will never eat yoghurt again!

This lasted about two weeks before I graduated to purified meals (stage 3 diet). Purified just means 'normal' meals liquidised, but they do not generally taste anything like the meal described on the plastic tray. I did not have a choice in the meal that arrived. It was often fish, because fish is a soft food, but I do not eat fish. Alas, I had no choice. Bizarrely, one of the best meals I had, which tasted like it said on the tray, was the much-maligned haggis. Seeing purified vegetables was strange: carrots, a blob of orange on the side of the plate, and peas, a bright green blob. I found I could not eat as much as I normally did, but I was eating again after eight weeks, and this was good. It was nice to feel food again in my mouth, and to drink coffee again was pure heaven. I had come a long way since June.

CHAPTER 7

Autumn Transition

The autumn air brushed against my face as I was wheeled on the stretcher through the automatic doors of the hospital to the ambulance wrapped like an Egyptian mummy. It was early September, and I was on my travels again. I was leaving the ARI after two and a half months, bound for the Neuro Rehab Unit (NRU) at Woodend Hospital.

Although I would spend double the time there, I was sad to leave neurology because everyone there was special to me, and the nursing staff had become good friends. As one nurse said, I was like one of the fittings! They gave me a leaving card signed by all of the nurses, something that apparently was unheard of before. I had come through a lot at the ARI, and it was relatively stress-free. Nevertheless, I was happy going to neuro rehab and the prospect of getting physiotherapy on my arms. I felt ready to move on.

The journey from one hospital to the next only took about fifteen to twenty minutes, but through the Aberdeen traffic, it seemed longer. As the ambulance entered the hospital grounds, I saw my new home for the first time. The granite buildings were pre-war and drab. Some of the buildings had glass structures on the frontage, modern add-ons that looked it. The ward was housed in the biggest building; to get to it we went through a set of sliding doors and to the right through a security locked door.

The ward was about thirty meters long by two meters wide, with a mix of single rooms and four-bed wards. I was put in a four-bed ward, though I was the only patient. My bed was at the back of the ward, right of two large bay windows that spanned the room end to end. It was a lovely view looking out onto the hospital grounds. A grassy area lay directly outside, in front of the window, with a beech tree to the right of my viewpoint. Shrubs were interspersed around the grassy lawn. A hedge separated the car park from the green area. Over the months, I would come to know this scene well while I watched the changing seasons. The hospital grounds were lined with beautiful mature trees that put on a spectacular free autumn show when their leaves changed into an array of colours from green to yellow to gold to red then finally to brown before they fluttered to the ground to carpet the grass.

The large bay windows offered a spectacular view when the blinds were opened in the mornings. I could see wildlife, rabbits feeding on the well-maintained grass and different breeds of dogs being walked among the grounds by visitors to the hospital.

The hospital was on the flight path to Aberdeen airport. Planes came into view at the top right of the window and made a gradual descent, losing about fifty feet, before I lost sight of them at the bottom left corner of the window. They were of different colours and sizes. One small plane was bright yellow. Over time I recognised various planes and what, I thought, they were used for. Planes with longer fronts, from the centre wheels to the nose, were long hauls, whereas shorter planes were used for domestic or European flights. I liked to imagine where the people had come from and whether their flight was for business or pleasure. In the mornings, from 7:00 a.m. onwards, things were a bit easier to deduce, as they were probably business people. Long hauls were a bit more difficult, but I would imagine their exotic destinations and the passengers on holidays . . . sunny cloudless blue skies and clear oceans . . . panoramic views of distant hills.

~w~

Distant Hills

Scotland's hills of towering majestic magnificence
Bring memories of wonderment and magnitude
Deceptively deceiving in their imposing splendour

Glencoe magnetically draws the brave and foolhardy

Osmotically drinking the atmosphere with every breath
Captivated with their impressive grandeur
Buachaille Etive Beag and Bidean nam Bian
Meal Dearg and Sgorr nam
Fiannaidh and Sgorr Dhearg and Sgorr Dhonuill
Guardians of secrets of a massacre century past

Climbers climb being mesmerised by beauty
Some triumph and some do not
And remain encapsulated in a world without end
Hills of tranquility and seductive elegance
Attractive appeal and deceiving deception
Geology often overcomes biological endeavours

—ᐤᠬᠬᠥ—

As the days passed, I settled into my new home. I had been assessed by the physiotherapists and given a manual wheelchair, which supported my back and legs. By this stage of my recovery, both arms were still sore, particularly the left shoulder, and I needed twenty-four-hour care, a nurse to feed me, and a sling to transfer into my wheelchair or shower chair. The nurses were all very nice and thought nothing of assisting me, but I never did and never will like people helping me. That is just my character. The wheelchair was self-propelling, but I needed someone to push it because I could not propel a wheelchair by myself whether it was manual or electric. In a few weeks I was assessed by the wheelchair service (MARS) and given a manual wheelchair of my own, a luxurious recliner.

In early December, I was assessed again for an electric wheelchair, but would have to wait some considerable time, as the list was long. At least I could operate an electric wheelchair, so this was a big improvement compared to a few months previously, when I could not even lift my arms let alone control a wheelchair.

CHAPTER 8

Nathan's Gift

I had been on the ward by myself for about a week or so when I got my first roommate, Nathan. His first question to me, as I was being fed by a nurse, was, "What's your favourite band?" I said Iron Maiden, and from that moment on, we were friends for life. My voice was still very soft and weak, but Nathan became so attuned to me that the nurses would ask him what I was saying. In just a few weeks, Nathan had become an expert in understanding me.

The ward played heavy metal music every morning and at various times throughout the day, including Iron Maiden, Metallica, Black Sabbath, and AC/DC. We were soon known as the Heavy Metal Ward. My musical education was expanding. Nathan taught electric guitar, and I absolutely loved it when he played. My dream had come true!

Nathan was such a kind person and a true friend. He let me watch programmes on his iPad, including musical performances and films. My arms were still useless, so Nathan always set up the iPad for me. He helped to feed me, thus freeing up the nurses, and he advised the hospital staff on the best place to position the buzzer. My hands did not have a lot of strength, though the right had a little more movement than the left, so I used a squeeze-ball type buzzer.

Nathan had a great sense of humour and was a brilliant storyteller. Sometimes I laughed so much that it hurt. Laughter helped me forget about my awful situation for a while. I laughed and laughed. Such fun times we had. I will never forget those magical days. We also enjoyed in-depth conversations on a variety of topics, from cellular biology to world politics. One afternoon we reminisced about children's programmes that were popular when we were growing up in the 1970s: The Magic Roundabout, Blue Peter, Bagpuss, Grange Hill, The Clangers, Tiswas, Crackajack, Multi-Coloured Swap Shop, Ivor the Engine, Jackanory, Rainbow, Vision On, The Banana Splits, Animal Magic, Andy Pandy, Record Breakers, The Muppet Show, Hector's House, Magpie, and Play School.

On another occasion, we came up with the idea of putting a sign on the wardrobe door labeled The Bad Boys Club. We made certain nurses honorary members, or anyone else who lived up to our very high standards. News of this exclusive club soon got around the ward and beyond, and people wanted to become members, such was the club's appeal.

As the weeks passed, I watched Nathan improve almost on a daily basis, as he graduated from a manual wheelchair to walking aids, and then to walking independently. I knew that I would soon lose my friend when it came time for him to depart the Heavy Metal Ward and return to the world outside the hospital. The day finally came when I had to say good-bye to him.

I will never forget Nathan.

CHAPTER 9

Getting Stronger

I received physiotherapy three times a week on my arms and legs. I also was allowed to use the Motomed, generally after a session. It was a bike for wheelchair users, but unlike a normal bike where you sit on a saddle, with the Motomed you sit in your chair to propel the pedals. A motor assists with pedaling, if required. My legs were strapped onto the pedals, and away I went. I could generally pedal for fifty minutes, though I often pedaled for more than an hour. Turning the top part around to face me exercised my arms in a circular motion. Over the weeks and months, my arms gradually improved and were not as sore. I did not need them resting on pillows, and they had more movement, though the right arm was more flexible than the left.

I still needed to be fed, and after several feedings, I made a funny observation: when someone is feeding you, they open their mouth just as they put the spoon into your mouth.

I was left-handed, so seeing my right arm improve was extremely frustrating. This improvement appeared to be exploited by the physiotherapists. They concentrated more on exercising the right than the left simply because it showed more improvement, or so it seemed, whereas to my reasoning, if the left was lagging, it should have received more attention.

This process is called neuroplasticity, where neuronal connections are made in the brain. However, I remonstrate, and it seemed to have worked for a while.

The physiotherapists were so kind and helpful as well as utterly professional. I will always be indebted to them. As the months passed, I did notice a slight improvement in my left arm, which continues to improve and will hopefully do so over time.

Now I could put a name to my shoulder condition. I had brachial plexus. The brachial plexus is a series of nerves formed by the anterior rami of the lower four cervical nerves. This plexus extends from the spinal cord through to the cervicoaxillary canal in the neck. No one can really say if I will make a good recovery or not, as this is the unknown factor.

Nevertheless, I cling to the hope I will. The doctors in the ARI, all these months previous, said I should, but it will take a year or so.

CHAPTER 10

Writing With My Eyes

November would prove to be a landmark month for me. I was still being fed through my PEG, as well as eating semi-normal food. I had been on a purified (stage 3) diet for six weeks – loving every mouthful! – after which I graduated to the next level, a soft diet. As the name implies, it is soft foods like corned-beef hash mashed down even more. As I managed to eat some 'real' food, the dietitian reduced the amount I was fed through my PEG, as well as the fluids (water). I was doing so well that by the middle of November, I was no longer getting anything via my PEG, and that was a wonderful feeling. It did mean I had to drink enough fluids myself, which was not a problem.

A week after being allowed to eat a soft diet, I graduated again to the next level, the final stage of this tiered system: a normal diet. I could eat anything within reason. I was left to decide what to eat. I found that rice stuck in my throat unless it was mixed with a sauce, so I avoided eating rice. I also avoided foods with crumbs, such as crumbles, as those too stuck in my throat. I will never forget nurse Arlene's facial expression of utter shock when I chose to eat a salad to show Linda, my speech-and-language therapist, that I was able to eat a normal solid diet. She cut up the various salad items into bite-size chunks to keep me from choking. Poor Arlene! I proved a point though. It felt good to be able to eat a normal diet again after five months.

Towards the end of the month, Speech and Language gave me a loan, as long as I was at Woodend Hospital, of a HeadMouse so I could use my laptop. My world suddenly widened. I could send emails for the first time in months. A HeadMouse is similar to a webcam in that a camera sits on top of the laptop screen and tracks eye movements. I wore glasses with the lens taken out so a sticky silver dot could be stuck on the bridge. By moving my eye-gaze, I was able to move the mouse across the screen. I could open a program by lingering my gaze on the icon for a couple of seconds.

As time went on, I became bored of doing nothing in particular on the laptop and needed mental stimulation. *I know*, I thought. *I'll write a book!* I was sure that I was not the only person to have suffered this condition and have gone through what I had experienced. Even if the book served as an incentive to encourage other people, it would have been worth writing. My writing time would be determined by the daily ward schedule and when I was showered and ready to face another day. I never asked the ward staff, "Can I get up so I can write?" Instead, I patiently waited my turn. It took two people to get me ready in the mornings. I would lie in bed thinking about what I was going to write and the phraseology. Sometimes I could only manage a couple hours writing, while at other times I was able to write for six hours. I started writing this book in Woodend Hospital using a HeadMouse, and completed about a third of the book whilst there, but finished it in Turner Memorial Hospital in Keith using an ordinary on-board keyboard, which everyone has. The book took about four months to finish. It was a slow arduous process. When the nurses and doctors found out what I was doing, they were most interested to see what I would say about them, but I assured them it was all good!

CHAPTER 11

Café Society

One of the buildings housed in the grounds of Woodend Hospital is the Royal Vulnerary Service (RVS) café. All the profits of the café go to the hospital. It is a circular building, and I had to go outside to get to it. Sitting there surrounded by windows, the views of the hospital grounds are spectacular. The café has about ten or so tables, and they also sell newspapers, magazines, books, sweets and essential toiletries. I was allowed to drink and eat by this time, so I visited the café with Mum and Dad as well as my sister and her husband. It sold good coffee and cakes, though one mouthful of Mum or Dad's cake filled me up. I looked forward to my café visits two or three times a week. I enjoyed the atmosphere of the place: patients with relatives, hospital workers buying snacks, or just members of the public buying coffee in an act of goodwill to show support for the hospital.

Sometimes upon leaving the café, my family took me for walks around the grounds. This was dependent on the weather, of course. Seeing the leaves changing colours from flaming reds to rustic browns and custardy yellows was exhilarating. When I left the neuro rehab ward in late January, I would miss my weekly visits to the café.

CHAPTER 12

Christmas in Neuro

I spent my first ever Christmas in hospital and felt lucky it was in the neuro rehab ward where I felt at home. Two weeks before Christmas, carol singers visited the ward to spread happiness and goodwill to all, singing seasonal songs with gusto. Most patients enjoyed them, and even the nurses sang along. I lay in bed singing "Run to the Hills" by Iron Maiden! Two Christmas trees were decorated at the front and back of the Day Room, a large room, measuring about 20 x 14 meters with windows lining two walls. In the summer months, it was very warm, but in the winter months, on frosty and snowy days, it was freezing cold. On a positive note, the windows offered magnificent views of the grounds, especially when the trees took on their autumn colours. In the far right corner, as you entered the room through a small passage, was a large flat-screen television.

On the opposite wall from the television was another flat-screen TV, which was used for Wii games such as ten-pin bowling. The Day Room was prominently used during mealtimes when patients, those who could get out of bed, sat at two oak circular tables. The oak wooden floor was beautiful. Over the months, I became very familiar with that room.

The Christmas tree lights twinkled at both ends of the room. Mr. Bean played on the television in the corner. The nurses and patients wore Christmas hats.

Tablecloths covered the tables, and bottles of soft drinks stood in the middle. A three-course meal was served for Christmas, but I could only eat two courses. I actually surprised myself with the amount I ate – turkey with all the trimmings followed by Christmas pudding with cream/custard or trifle.

Christmas Day was pleasant and good spirited. The ward put on a very good show, but I still felt sad because I could not be with my mum. The ward gave every patient a Christmas present, which was extremely nice of them and very much appreciated.

I also spent New Year in the neuro rehab ward. Hogmanay was a low-key affair with "The Bells," for me anyway, non-eventful. I was asleep! I hoped, when I awoke in the morning, that 2018 would be better than 2017. It could not get much worse!

CHAPTER 13

Missing the Thrill of Driving

I knew I would be moving on from the neuro rehab ward within a few weeks, or at least by the end of the month. A date had been set, some weeks before, for my PEG to be removed on Thursday, 11th January, 2018. I could not wait.

I remembered when it was put into my stomach and how ill I was coughing up blood and needing to be taken to theatre. The night before I was due to go to the ARI for the PEG removal, I had to fast, since this was a medical procedure. Wrong, as it turned out. I was not allowed breakfast, not even a drink. The patient transport ambulance arrived not long after I had been washed. I was wrapped like an Egyptian mummy and placed onto the stretcher. An auxiliary, Shannon, who was doing her nurse training, accompanied me. The stretcher was fastened to the floor of the ambulance, and when all were aboard, we were off on the fifteen-minute journey. It was a nice sunny January day. Upon arriving at the ARI, I was wheeled to the ward where the PEG would be removed and transferred to a bed. My appointment was at 11:00 a.m., and the doctor arrived at about 11:30 am. It only involved cutting the tube and pushing the small bung, smaller than a pinky fingertip, into the stomach to be expelled naturally. The whole thing took two minutes. We waited about twenty minutes for the ambulance to arrive for the return journey. From leaving the ward to returning to the ward took three hours for a two-minute procedure. I was so hungry when I returned that I ate two Weetabix and drank a mug of coffee.

As I lay in the hospital bed earlier that morning, a horrible thought occurred to me: *I might never drive again.* This thought, it has to be said, was the bitterest pill to swallow of all that I have had to deal with since this awful nightmare started. I felt so desperately sad that I was close to tears. The thought of not being able to drive again, not getting behind a steering wheel, was so over-bearing that I couldn't imagine the awful prospect. Some people don't like driving and give it up voluntarily, but the pleasure and freedom of driving was taken away from me in a cruel, ten-second, silly accident. Driving was not just important in my life for getting the shopping and running errands. It was more than that. I loved being in the car. I often went driving just out of sheer enjoyment. As with the case of so many things that have been taken from me, driving was another cruel blow. How I loved driving my VW

Caddy, my sixth car, but by far the best. My dad had adapted it for me, and that made it even more special.

The reality of this loss hit me full force. Never again would I hear the air compressor as the back door lifted, the lowering of the ramp and the squeaking of the electric wheelchair tyres as it went up. Never again would I experience the thrill of cruising down the carriageway hearing the null sound of the tyres on the road and the soothing, rhythmic sound of the engine. I loved driving along local coast roads, seeing and smelling the sea as it lapped onto the yellow sands. It was like watching white horses disappear as they galloped to shore. Blue skies on a summer's day with cotton-ball clouds floating overhead...the salty air hitting your nostrils...driving to Inverness or Aberdeen for day outings.

In Inverness, I would have coffee, wander around the shops and go to the cinema. I could do everything myself, and that was the best part. How I would miss the thrill of driving down the A9 (Scotland's main artery) to Perth, and gazing at the beautiful scenery of the Highlands while driving south. The joy of zigzagging winding roads was wonderfully thrilling. I am not one of those people who go to car shows or drool over fancy sport cars, happy merely to admire them. No, I want to drive them! Sometimes I have a wild and crazy desire to drive a car transporter full of Lamborghinis as fast as I can go and then crash. Look at the damage I could do! On second thought, maybe it's a good thing I can't drive anymore!

I have never been one for going abroad, spending the majority of your holiday in an airport, probably because it was such a nightmare organising everything. Besides, I couldn't give a jot seeing foreign climes when there's such beauty in Scotland, from the outstanding magnificent scenery of the Highlands to the rolling hills of the Borders and everywhere in between. I would like to explore Scotland in a specially adapted campervan. How wonderful that would be! My idea of total utopia, but that dream will never become reality, as a campervan like that would be horrendously expensive. I couldn't afford a tyre let alone the van.

I have absolutely no time for those people who say disabled shouldn't drive, and spuriously put forward nonsensical arguments to back up their claim. I suspect some say this because they see us as perpetually simplistic children. If you have passed a driving test, you have as much right to be on the road as they have, and one could argue possibly more right because your freedom is limited otherwise, something they never have to experience.

I might, however, be able to drive again, but the adaptations would be very expensive, as well as maintaining the vehicle, and I could not afford the car/van.

What I wouldn't give to drive again, but those are distant memories of happy times gone.

I have two ambitions in my life, but whether I will ever achieve them, I do not know. They are to drive again, to feel the freedom of the open road, and to live in my beautiful Fochabers independently. I was so pleased when I passed my driving test, and enjoyed driving my different cars.

After passing my driving test and relishing my newfound freedom, I needed to think about my next challenge: driving solo. Well I remember the excitement and nervousness my first time driving alone with noone in the passenger's seat to tell me what to do. I decided that I wanted to learn more about the techniques of driving, so I took the Advanced driving test. This test teaches you how to drive safely and to your own capabilities. It teaches you how to read the road and anticipate what might happen and avoid anything that could pose a danger to you. They require you to give a running commentary during my test, which I took with an Advanced Driving police driver. At one point, I said, "On the grass verge to my right-hand side is a dead rabbit!" Maybe too much detail, but alas, I passed the test the first time with flying colours and became the first wheelchair user in Moray to do so.

Now, that thrill, that boyish excitement, has gone from my life, probably forever, lost in the blink of an eye. This horrible ordeal, which I would not wish on anyone, has robbed me of what I spent forty years achieving. I gave up smoking and drinking because the car always came first. I used to weigh the cost – cigarettes or petrol – and petrol always won. Eighteen years ago I said goodbye to alcohol, as drinking and driving do not go together, and the car was far more important than drinking would ever be, so the car won again.

I get annoyed when I hear on the news or read in the papers about people being one-seven times over the drink-drive limit. If you drive, then you should not touch a drop of alcohol, or even eat a piece of cake with alcohol in it. Don't they know what they have? Don't they know how easily that freedom can be lost? It is something I can only dream about now.

CHAPTER 14

Next Stop: Moray

The January chill felt cold on my face as I left the neuro rehab ward five months after the ambulance's stretcher wheeled me through the sliding doors on a hot September day. One of my favourite nurses kissed my cheek before she stood and waved goodbye. As the patient ambulance pulled away from the pre-war buildings that comprise the stately Woodend Hospital, memories came flooding back: Nathan, who I will never forget for the music and laughter; Bob's magnetic character; my first Christmas spent in hospital; walking over to the RVS café.

During the months I spent in NRU, the nursing staff became friends as well as medics and carers. This is not a book about nurses and doctors, but the NRU meant so much to me that I have to mention some of the medical staff who touched my life, made me laugh and comforted me in bad times. I cannot remember everyone. Sister Laura, whose soothing, bedside manner was so reassuring – such a lovely person. Every time I eat an orange, I'll think of Laura. I'll never forget Susan, who brightened my day every time she came on duty, and made me laugh when she fed me. Then there's the infamous Ziggy, who kept me laughing with his off-the-wall sense of humour and our sensible conversations. Nicky was definitely one of my favourites, with her compassion and loving-kindness. Clare, sweet Clare, would lighten my days with her kindness and humility. This poem is for you, Clare, inspired by a conversation we had about the *Mona Lisa*.

-ᗯᒍᐯ-

Lady with the Mystic Smile

People moved to the side, parting of the waves
Shuffles to leave a clear passage
"Let the wheelchair through," security said
Symbol of recognisable difference
A chariot, unknowing announcement and simplicity

Da Vinci's *Mona Lisa* still draws magnetically
Osmotically drinking in the
Lady's smile and charisma
Shrouded mystery of her true identity fascinates
Who is she? What was the connection?
Centuries roll and theories mount, but no definitive
A series of possibilities adds to the conundrum

The Louvre, right of the Seine, home to *Mona Lisa*
How far removed from Italy and her lifestyle
Now being spied upon in a conspicuous capital
Solitary hanging for all to admire and marvel
Small in presence though tall in popular recognition
Eyes following in an act of compulsive observation

—w~—

I will always remember Linda's refreshing to-the-point way of speaking and *Happy Days* catch phrase. How can I ever forget Australian Wendy's kindness and beauty? I hope, one day, that "We'll Meet Again." Dr. Gooday's kind and lovely bedside manner made everything a little bit bearable. Lorraine was a special person. Elaine and Pam's sensibility was extremely welcome. Chelsea touched me with her kindness and humility, as well as with her deep, heartfelt story. Carol, the ward's caretaker, was so good about feeding me so the nurses could do other things; as sister Laura would say, "My Daily Date."

I'm so thankful to Marion, ward receptionist, who also fed me and told me stories about her interesting life. Angelika, who I instantly took to, became my favourite because of her calming manner and the way she spoke directly to people. Something about her soothing Polish accent and kind humility really touched my heart. She was an excellent student nurse and will be an outstanding staff nurse. I miss seeing Angelika.

As we headed out of Aberdeen, I saw a Baxter's lorry heading south full of food products, destined for far-off markets. Nostalgic memories flooded back of my beloved Fochabers. I started to feel deeply sad at the prospect of not seeing the River Spey again.

—ₘₘ—

The Spey

Majestic sounds of the water flowing past
Streaming over rocks in a fluidity of forcefulness
Salmon leaping on their migratory journey
Canoes weave their way to their destination

I sit in reflective solitude
My beloved Spey soothes and washes and cleanses
Picturesque vistas and flowing, restores neural calmness
The waters inspire as well as rejuvenate
Neural synaptic connections intertwine galvanised
thought processes
My beloved Spey swirls and surges on its journey
unaware of its comforting tranquility

—ₘₘ—

The journey north was nice, gazing at trees in their winter bareness; ploughed fields lying dormant on the surface, but active under the frozen soil; distant cattle and sheep grazing the almost grassless fields, searching for nutrition from patches around them before moving on; the yellow-cold sun sinking down the sky, a visible reminder that it was still January. I was glad to see the sign that announced 'Welcome to Moray.' I was almost home. It was time for the next stage in my recovery.

CHAPTER 15

Months Become a Year

Arriving at Turner Memorial Hospital in Keith, I was apprehensive, as I did not know what to expect. I did know, however, that this would be the last hospital before moving on. Keith is a small town in the North-East of Scotland, about fifty miles north of Aberdeen. It is a friendly place where people speak to each other. There is a nice sense of community, and people look out for one another rather than living in their own small bubble, isolating themselves.

The hospital is situated just off the main street and has about twenty beds, three wards of four, as well as seven single rooms. I was in a single room other than a couple of nights in one of the wards.

It was a rehab hospital, and I particularly enjoyed my times on the Motomed looking out the window at the beech tree and listening to Radio 3, watching the clouds floating across the sky, winds swaying the twigs on the tree, and the sun brightening the distant landscapes.

There was also a Day Room, but not as big as the one at Woodend, where most of the patients went for meals, relaxing or just to watch television. On the far wall hung a painting of Lossiemouth, the hometown of my friend Ron, my second roommate at Woodend. He followed me from Woodend Hospital to Turner Memorial in Keith. When someone has experienced all that Ron and I went through, it cements a lasting bond. He is a kind man with humility, and very patient. Poor Ron had to endure heavy metal music as well as Nathan's and my silliness, but he took it in stride. Coming roughly from the same neck of the woods (North-East Scotland), we had a commonality. We got on well, and we both spent Christmas in hospital. Ironically, or by design, we both ended up moving to the same sheltered housing complex.

As the weeks passed, my left arm regained sufficient movement that I could use an ordinary hand-held mouse on the laptop. My increased arm movement could be attributed to the physiotherapy exercises, particularly Christine's inventive abilities.

This made a significant difference in that I had more control. I used the on-screen keyboard and became quite good with it. I found, over time, that I became quite adept at finding the various keys. I enjoyed Turner Memorial, and the staff were very friendly.

By this point I had been in hospitals for nine months, so I just wanted my freedom and a semblance of normality in my life. Time to move on and find out what life had in store. Spring was just around the corner, and I yearned to feel the sun on my face and to enjoy long summer days.

CHAPTER 16

The Loss of Everything

As I write this in June of 2018, I am still in hospital awaiting discharge. I have been in hospitals over a year now. I have been in Keith Turner Memorial five months longer than I should have been. I am bed blocking, one of 20,000-plus, and that is totally shocking. The frustrating part is not being able to restart my life after all this time. Another totally shocking part is knowing that because I am not a medical patient, I'm denying a patient a bed who does have medical needs.

I gave back my house to the Council (end of my tenancy 26 June, 2018) after seventeen years because it was unsuitable for my wheelchair. Losing my house was first suggested a few months earlier, and I just wanted the ground to open up and swallow me. I wanted to die at the thought of never going back, but that is what happened.

My life has been turned upside down and will never be the same again.

Looking from the kitchen window at my neighbour's Japanese Acer tree and the beautiful rhododendron bush with crimson flowers in the summer … sitting in the back garden listening to the slow flow of the Foch Burn … lost memories, gone in the blink of an eye.

-ᴡᴍ-

Japanese Acer

Shrouded in oriental mystical past
Mountain maple grows uninhibited skyward
Looking elegant covered in a deep red bark

The cold frosty days of winter the Acer illuminates
Joyously lighting up the long dreary days
In an act of steadfastly urban sophistication

Symbiosis from the other plants seems to encourage
Prompting and supporting and inspiring
Allied champion of other forms of nature to survive

Birds shelter and rest and forage for sustaining food
Insects single-mindedly scurry on their life cycle

From my window I watch the seasonal changes
Spring heralds rebirth of buds and nutritional growth

Summer sees an efflorescence array of bloom
Autumn the windswept cascading waterfall of leaves
Winter bareness in readiness to start the cycle again

⎯ⱽⱽⱽ⎯

I hope I will be rehoused, and truly hope it is back to my beloved Fochabers, though I doubt I will ever live there again. I love Fochabers so I feel like a Fochaberian. I had to leave the village three times in seventeen years for an extended period, and the pain I felt was unbearable in my eagerness to get back home again. Now I will never go back 'home' to my house nor probably to Fochabers, and it hurts so much. Everyone keeps saying how unsuitable the house was and how I won't be going back there. I wanted to cry at the thought of not going back to Christie Place again. No one understands! They humour me by saying that I will get a house in Fochabers again, but they know my days of living independently are over, and that makes me even sadder.

Making a mug of coffee first thing in the morning … going on the bike twice/three times a day … sitting in the kitchen with my back against the fridge listening to the radio … sitting in the back garden listening to the crows in the trees on summer mornings as the Foch Burn flows behind the fence on its way to the Spey … opening the kitchen blinds in the morning to welcome the day, and closing them at night … sitting at the front door on summer mornings enjoying the warm sunshine on my face … shutting the blinds in the sitting room and bedrooms on hot summer days to keep the rooms cool … speaking on the intercom when the doorbell rang, and opening the door if I recognised the voice … doing my own clothes washing … filling the dishwasher. All these memories, and many more, are gone and will never return.

I do not particularly like the fact that I am in no-man's land, not knowing what is going to happen next, not being in control of my life. I'm caught between a rock and a hard stone.

I lived in Fochabers for seventeen years without feeling in danger or threatened once. Maybe I only deserve to be happy for seventeen years while others live their own lives unimpeded.

I have no money and as a result cannot afford an adapted house, physiotherapy, and 24-hour care, so consequently I have to let others decide my future. I am not in charge of my destiny, and that frightens me, and makes me feel vulnerable. The feeling of uncertainty is extremely terrifying.

I have lost so much that I wonder was it all worth it? I am lucky, they say, in a 'could be worse' voice. Really? How much worse? My arms will never again work quite as well as before my accident. I cannot lift a cup of water to my mouth to drink, feed myself, use a smart-phone (like most, I did virtually everything on my phone before my accident), sign my name or even wipe my nose when I sneeze. I have lost my house, and I will never live independently again. I must be dependent on people for my personal care and to dress me and hoist me in and out of my wheelchair.

They say every cloud has a silver lining, but it is well hidden so far, and any positives have not revealed themselves.

Ten seconds changed my life in so many ways that I wonder if my life was ruined in that brief span of time.

CHAPTER 17

Disabled Body, Able Brain

Sometimes it feels like I have become a non-entity who should conform to society's anachronistic perceptions that if you're physically disabled, you need to be locked away in "a safe environment" and have lots of social contact in case you become anti-social overnight and become a "vulnerable adult" (a term I hate). The prospect of living independently, living my life according to me, is seen as bad. Horrible things *might* happen, but most likely will not.

This perceived fear factor is executed using dodgy psychology and the fear-of-God tactic. I'm sick of being humoured as if I'm a child who cannot see through the simplicity.

I'm required to have someone who has Power of Attorney over me in case I cannot perform a certain task like signing my name or, as I suspect, have not the mental ability to decide. But may I state emphatically that I have a physical ailment, not a cognitive condition. A physical disability does not necessarily mean a cognitive problem, but sadly, cynically, I would say, society often makes the link between physical disability and cognitive impairment.

How graciously society bestows accolades!

I agree everyone should have Power of Attorney in place in case of unforeseen eventualities, but this should not be seen as a controlling mechanism. I will decide when, and to whom, this legal instrument will be put into place.

Come on, please! I am going to be a doctor of neuroscience, so do not insult me or play mind games.

What keeps me going is returning to my Open University studies and earning my PhD. Over the years, I have studied a number of courses, mostly in human biology, with the Open University. The course that proved most useful in the hospital environment was the MSc course in medicinal chemistry, with the utterly fantastic Dr. Kay.

-vvv-

Open University

Educator of the masses without societal barriers
All coming together in a common unity
Society's class statuses hold no governing rule
Instead passion and enthusiasm and eagerness
Advancement and achievement and pride objectives
Giving hope to the dejected and dreams to dreamers

In a voyage of discovery to explore unforeseen worlds

The OU largest educator of disabled
Societal barriers of preconceptions
Imbecilic condescending supercilious chains are broken

My beloved OU is there in dark and joyous times
Non-judgmental of physical imperfections
Neural achievements are the only criteria
A constant when life becomes overbearing
Access with no barriers and an addicted student
True equality and not just meaningless sound bites

Opportunity of sameness is refreshing in its parity
No diminishing of educational standards
Same TMAs and EMAs exasperated expectations
Same frustrating neural stress and pleasurable thrill
Equality at its finest with no barriers

In a world of uncertainty and fakery
The OU is a shining light to show the way
Few can follow the leader though try but fail
Educator of the masses and destroyer of myths
Restoring confidence and hope to ultimate success

꧁꧂

CHAPTER 18

New Horizons

It has been eighteen months since my accident on that fateful June morning, 2017. My life, as I knew it then, has totally changed beyond all recognition. Friends I have made in the sheltered housing complex where I live now see me as someone who is reliant on others to do everything for him: preparing meals, feeding, giving drinks through a straw, giving personal care, switching on the TV, wiping a hair from my eye, wiping my nose when I sneeze, scratching my eyebrow when it's itchy. They never knew the fiercely independent person I was for fifty years; instead, all they've known is this shell of a man who cannot do anything for himself. I even have to rely on others to open a door for me, a simple, basic task.

I spent a total of thirteen months in four hospitals before being discharged. Following my discharge from hospital, the authorities did not know where to place me, as there were no places for younger disabled like me – a stressful and totally shocking situation to be in. People and/or government bodies should hang their heads in shame at this lack of provision for young disabled. (Does anyone really care?) I moved into a sheltered housing complex 30th July 2018, which provides 24-hour care. The complex is a safe, secure environment in that people who enter or leave the building are monitored. There are thirty individual flats over two levels, and I have my own flat on the ground level. All the flats surround a central courtyard so that the fifteen flats on the upper level look down on the landscaped garden, while those on the lower level look out over the spectacular array of multi-coloured flowers and plants in the summer.

It is a new building, and I am very lucky to have been offered a flat, but I still long to move back to Fochabers one day. Sadly, I do not think my dream of waking in the morning seeing The Spey flow past is a realistic one. I have this recurring dream of having lots of money so I can build a big, specially adapted house over-looking The Spey, driving my own customized adapted van, and employing 24-hour care. Now, that would be nice!

Everyone is so kind to me here, from tenants to the care staff, and we all have a good laugh. I have a special rapport with the carers, as they have to do everything for me. I have one of the highest care requirements in the place, not something I am proud about. Going from almost total independence to needing 24-hour care is a big adjustment as well as self-degrading.

People say that they can understand or imagine what it's like for me. No, they cannot! Unless, you experience something like this, you cannot imagine what it feels like to be physically unable to do anything. Losing power in your arms must be the worst thing that can happen to a person, and for a wheelchair user, it is catastrophic.

I moved into the same complex as my good friend Ron; in fact, he is only one flat away. Ron and I spent six months in hospitals together. We have a special bond because we experienced a lot during the same period in our lives.

I got an electric wheelchair with a tray in front where the controller is fixed. It is a lovely chair, and I thank the Wheelchair Service (MARS) for giving me it. I can regularly be seen zooming around the complex or to the shops. Being unable to lift a cup to my mouth means I have to keep myself hydrated. I bought a water bottle and have it attached to the back of my wheelchair.

What does the future have in store? I do not know! I would never have predicted eighteen months ago that I would be in sheltered housing needing 24-hour care. But that is exactly what happened. To say I never get low and say 'Why me?' would not be true, but I try not to show my feelings.

Recently, The Open University (OU) honoured me by hosting a Graduation Ceremony. The Director of The OU in Scotland, MSP, Minister for Education in

Scotland, family and friends, as well as tenants and staff at the complex were all there. It was particularly good to see my lovely neighbour from Fochabers, Charlie. Without Charlie and his wife Ninnie's intervention on that fateful day, I wouldn't be here today.

I like living in this complex and have been made so welcome, but this painful hankering to live in Fochabers again won't go away and never will until I'm back there. In reality, however, I don't think I will ever live in Fochabers again, and that cold fact hurts so much. I have to make do with the hand I'm dealt, however much I want a change. I am too disabled and need a lot of help, and that's the determining factor. Sure, I will be humoured and spoken to like I'm a child, in a subtly psychological way, but the fact still remains that I will always want to move back to Fochabers however much I am spoken imbecilically to by those who think they know better.

It makes me so deeply sad that I will never drive again. People are too matter-of-fact about what driving meant to me. "Not the end of the world, is it!" To me it is, pal! If I had the money, I would have a campervan specially adapted to my needs so I could tour my lovely Scotland.

I have lost so much over the past eighteen months, from my independence to romantic aspirations. I have become another meaningless statistic in a bureaucratic society! I do not have money, which could have opened doors, as money does, and could have paid for intensive physiotherapy at the appropriate time, when it might have helped. A so-called professional insinuated recently that I had regained all mobility "that they thought I would." A similar thing was said to my parents eighteen months ago as I lay in hospital with a ventilating tube down my throat, by a consultant who thought I wouldn't survive the night, but I proved them wrong with my fierce will to live as independently and as well as possible.

I exercise my arms on my own, and my dad comes in every day to put me on my exercise machine. Since I have started exercising, I can see that my left arm, the arm most affected, is showing more improvement than the right. Being a left-hander, I am very happy to see that improvement.

Whilst lying in Intensive Care, one thing kept me going above all others. That something was returning to my studies with the Open University. I wrote and published an article on the topic of Cerebral Palsy for OpenLearn, and in January 2019, I applied to study for my PhD. With determination and diligent study, it will be a successful endeavour.

I look forward and not backward, and I approach each new day with a positive attitude and a sense of humour and delight in the beauty of the world. Thank you for reading my book. I hope it has touched your life, encouraged you, and inspired you. If you are struggling, please know that you are not alone. Reach out to anyone in your life who may be able to help. Most of the time, you will find a hand reaching back toward you to lift you up in your time of need.

A Note From the Author

I live in the North-East of Scotland in a sheltered housing complex. Since my accident, my life is totally different to what it was before, in that I have lost my independence and have to rely on other people to help me with everything.

I enjoy a full and active life. One of my favourite hobbies is playing chess. I'm not very good at it, but I enjoy the mind warfare. I also enjoy listening to music, and I appreciate a wide spectrum of musical genres and styles, from classical to heavy metal.

I have been an Open University student for twenty-six years and have three degrees in science. I earned my MSc a few months before being admitted to Intensive Care, and am currently working toward earning my PhD.

The purpose of my book *Ten Seconds That Changed My Life* is to put forward a disabled person's perspective and to encourage those who are differently abled to persevere no matter what challenges they may face.

Feel free to email me at: tensecondslife@gmail.com. I would love to hear from you.

If you enjoyed this book and it touched your life in some way, I would appreciate a great review on Amazon. Thank you!

Iain MacLeod